Praise for

Jackisms:

Weight Loss Humor and Help from My Weight Losing Friends

"When Jack walked through the door of my Weight Watchers meeting (now called WW workshop), he brought a new energy with him that has helped many WW members remember his important pieces of advice by boiling them down to "Jackisms." This book is not only a great collection of "Jackisms," but also an application to Alexandra's life in a very practical way. In sharing some of her weight loss struggles, Alexandra has also helped me to focus on the three most important things in our ongoing battle to get healthy: acceptance of oneself, patience for the eventual outcome, and perseverance to keep going even in tough times. Yes, I might have lost 158 pounds on WW, but I also look to people sitting in the chairs around me at my WW Workshop for inspiration. Alexandra and Jack are two such people whose words of inspiration resonate with me and who I appreciate weekly!"

    ----**Cheryl Harris-Sumida**,
       Theater Coach, Librarian, 10-year member of WW,
       lost 158 pounds on WW

"These bits of wisdom made me smile, nod in agreement, and have an "aha!" moment or two! Some also made me stop and think about where I am in my own weight loss journey. This book would be a great gift for someone just starting the WW program as well as for someone who has been in it for awhile. You might even consider gifting it to yourself!"

    ----**Emily Duerfeldt**, Retired Academic Advisor,
       lost 40 pounds on WW

Jackisms

Weight Loss Humor and Help from My Weight Losing Friends

ALEXANDRA GEORGAS

and Jack Demirgian, Cheryl Sumida, Jeff Carrillo, Judy, Donna, Susan, Carla Printz, Crystal Graves, Joe Suhayda, Margie McCarthy, Jodie Needham, and Louann

Jackisms:
Weight Loss Humor and Help from My Weight Losing Friends

By Alexandra Georgas

© Copyright 2019 Alexandra Georgas

ISBN 978-0-578-66488-0

Published by

Alexandra Georgas

www.alexandrageorgas.com

Table of Contents

Introduction

I have been attending Weight Watchers weekly meetings since 2001. Meetings tend to be attended mostly by women, and most people do not keep attending over the long term. Many lose their weight, quit, and show up again when the weight comes back on.

Then there is Jack. Jack reached his goal of 50 pounds lost on Weight Watchers in 2000. He not only has kept it off for the last 19 years, he has come to meetings the entire time, and usually attends two meetings a week.

Jack both inspires and entertains. I started jotting down what he said in meetings just to motivate myself. Then I realized he truly has some unique and humorous ways of putting things. I hope as you read what I call "Jackisms" you will both laugh and be motivated to take better care of yourself. I know I have.

1

Jack's story

One day while Jack was on vacation in Florida, he witnessed a middle-aged, overweight man drop dead right in front of him. The look of shock and pain on the faces of the man's wife and children jolted Jack. Jack was also a middle-aged, overweight man. Jack's father had passed away from a heart attack at age 62, his mother passed away from the same fate at age 63, and his grandfather died at age 60, also from a heart attack. Jack knew he would very likely have the same fate as his family and this Florida man if he didn't take action.

After returning home from vacation, Jack went to the post office to collect the mail he had accumulated. He dumped it out on his kitchen counter, and on top of the pile was a coupon to try Weight Watchers. He had never gotten one of those before, or since. He joined.

Before losing his weight, Jack used to host chocolate parties, where each person would bring their favorite chocolate and everyone would rate it. He still is a huge chocolate lover and even ate his favorite candy bars while losing his weight. Weight Watchers taught him how to eat what he loves, but in smaller amounts and by adding the healthy foods our bodies need. He proudly wears pro-chocolate T-shirts to Weight Watchers meetings, giving us a guaranteed chuckle.

Jack has a PhD in analytical chemistry from the State University of New York at Buffalo. After working as a chemist at the Argonne National Laboratory, he retired to enjoy time with his wife, children, and especially his five grandchildren. He also enjoys hiking, participating in Toastmasters, making his own T-shirts, attending Weight Watchers meetings, and of course, eating chocolate.

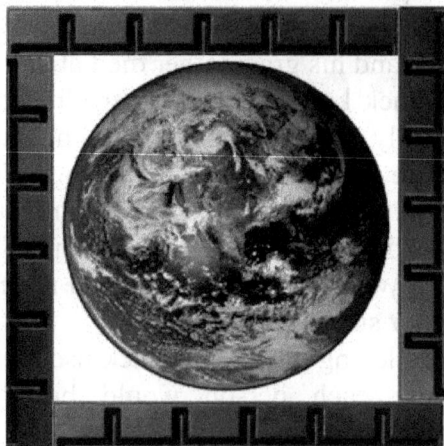

T-shirt design by Jack

Jackisms

Quotes from Jack

New Beginnings

"Tomorrow is a new day. It's a blank page."

When I was in college, after I lost 70 pounds on Weight Watchers the first time, I found myself struggling to stay on the program. One day as I sat in the common area of my dorm, trying to memorize facts as I prepared for a final, the vending machine started whispering to me. "Come. Come hither. I have nice treats to relieve your stress." I succumbed and ate a highly forbidden chocolate bar. Back then, the program didn't allow for candy, along with many other foods. Oh my, was that indulgence good. The metal machine spoke again: "Wasn't that fantastic? Don't you want to feel that great taste on your tongue again?" Yes, I partook. And partook again, and again. I finally stopped after the seventh candy bar. I left the scene of my sins and hid from the crime in my dorm room, feeling shocked at my binge, guilty, and a lot worse emotionally. The next day I didn't feel physically well, and to this day, unlike Jack, I really don't like to eat chocolate bars.

That binge could have turned into a week of rebellion. But I chose to get back on program and move forward. Years later, I heard Jack say after a member shared a similar experience in a meeting, "Tomorrow is a new day. It's a blank page." The next day's tracking journal pages are empty. The previous day's binge is not there on the next day's page. We truly can start again. One of my Weight Watchers leaders phrased this as, "You can get back on program as soon as you brush the crumbs off your face." So, let's. Forgive, and start anew.

Eat What You Love

"Use your points on foods you love."

In my younger years, when trying to lose weight I gave up eating many foods I loved and tried to eat "diet" foods, such as cottage cheese, fat-free cheese, and air-popped popcorn, all of which I don't really like. Then when I came across one of my favorite foods, I had a hard time not diving in and overindulging.

Jack's wise point is to actually do the opposite. Eat what you love and not what you don't love. That's the beauty of the modern Weight Watchers program: no foods are forbidden. We just have a points budget and have the freedom to choose what to eat. Jack lost his weight eating a chocolate bar every week. Instead of saying "no" to all the foods you love, budget some points to have them, but within your daily limits. Enjoy what you love, and you can lose weight and keep it off for life.

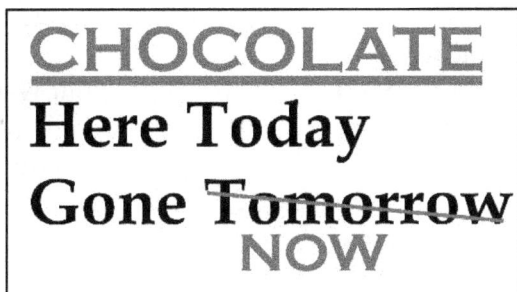

CHOCOLATE
Here Today
Gone ~~Tomorrow~~
NOW

T-shirt design by Jack

Water

"Drink more water because you get exercise by going to the bathroom."

When the body does not have enough water, a bunch of bad stuff happens. First, it spends energy trying to get water instead of doing things we want, like burning off some unwanted fat. Second, it holds on to whatever water it has, causing a water weight gain, which isn't so fun. Third, it sends signals to your brain saying, "Eat, eat, you need food" because it is smart enough to know there is water in a lot of foods, but dumb enough to think you will eat those types of foods when you are hungry. The body will also tell you to rest, giving you tiredness signals, to conserve what you have. So then you don't feel like doing anything, and that is bad too.

Now, purists will say to drink pure water with nothing in it; others like their water infused with fruit. Yes, sure, pure water is the healthiest, so if you can go that route, do it. But if you are a purist, could you please not preach about it in Weight Watchers meetings and kind of put down people who would rather have some better flavor in their liquids? Artificial sweeteners are not prohibited on Weight Watchers. Neither is diet soda. So if that's how we get our water, let us, folks. It's better to get it in via these methods than not drink at all. I've lost over 70 pounds (multiple times now) drinking diet soda. So, kids, hate to say it, but it's not that bad. Yes, it can give you false munchies, so watch how it makes you feel. And yes, you are taking in fun stuff that isn't actually adding nutrition, like the bubbles and flavorings. But if it helps you get in liquids, Weight Watchers wisely says, "You may partake."

We can live for weeks without food. We can only live a few days without water. Think about that. The body has to have it to live, and it will screw up your weight loss efforts if it is denied. So, enjoy!

Goal Setting

"You have to keep setting goals. Otherwise the dark side will call you back."

Once Jack reached his goal weight, in order to keep the weight off, he set new goals. One goal was to be able to hike the Grand Canyon. He trained hard and accomplished that goal.

I set a goal to be able to walk the 1.3 miles each way to and from my new job. At first it was painful and difficult, but I pressed on, and after a couple of weeks, not only could I do the walk, but my jeans were looser.

I set another goal to do my sticker motivation system. Every day if I track 100% I get a sticker for the day. If in addition I am under my daily points, I get a second sticker for that day. If I also add activity to that day, I get a third sticker. I find this daily little reward system helps me to stay on plan and do the program. After a while the stickers got to be routine, and so I added the reward that if I received so many stickers, I would allow myself to have pizza for dinner one night the next week. It's good to keep setting new goals, with new rewards. That keeps us motivated and making progress.

Calorie and Work Out Tracking

Lost 1 LB For The week

Points Goal per day: **34**   Calorie Goal per day: **1800**   Fat Gram Goal per day: **50**   Activity Points Goal per Day: **8**

Week: 12	Saturday	Sunday	Monday	Tuesday	Wednesday	Thursday	Friday	
Starting Weight Number (last digit only)	3	3	2	1	2	2	1	2
Total Points Consumed for the Day	48	43	51	47	49·	49	31	
Total Calories	2367	2010	2071	1685	1745		1802	
Total Fat Grams	105	75	69	51	59		80	
Gain/Loss	0	-1	-1	+1	0	-1	+1	
Tracked 100%?	A+	FANTASTIC!	GREAT!	AMAZING!	WOW!	GREAT!	WOW!	
Stayed under Max Calorie/Points Goal?				AMAZING!	WOW!		FANTASTIC!	
Stayed under Max Fat Gram Goal?				GREAT!				
Activity Done?	AMAZING!		SUPER!			AMAZING!	FANTASTIC!	
Activity Points Earned	31		22			12	25	
What Activity?	1 hour Golf lesson & 9 holes of Golf		Golfed 9 holes			1 hour Bowling lesson	walked in Gordens 1½ hrs Bowled 3 hrs.	
Emotions or Major Influencers	too much after dinner	Better after dinner. ☺	planned better fer snacks	massage + pedicure too many pretzels!		Tracked until big party at dinner		

My Sticker Sheet Invention

10

Alcohol Humor #1

"I cut my drinking in half. I only use one hand."

For the most part, I stay away from alcohol because I'm always trying to lose weight and I know alcohol interferes with weight loss. Drinking slows the entire system, including metabolism, so it is harder to lose weight. But over the years I've heard many a Weight Watchers member confess in meetings how they just love their favorite beer or wine or once in a while indulging in margaritas. And these are people who I observe are losing weight. How do they do it? Points budgeting. They plan for their favorite drinks. And they limit how many they have. Those who say "yes" to the drinks they love, but learn how to have these within limits, do lose weight. Learning to enjoy what we love and yet not overdoing it means a lifestyle we can maintain for the rest of our lives. So enjoy that drink. Just count it!

Enjoy Food

"If you are not emotionally satisfied with your meal, you will keep eating."

When we eat a meal with foods we really don't like or portions that are too small to satisfy, we will often end up rummaging around the kitchen not long after the meal is over. We may end up consuming too much for the day as a result. It is better to eat foods we really enjoy and in enough volume that we feel emotionally satisfied. Then after-meal snacking is not as large a challenge. If we try to lose weight by eating foods that do not satisfy, we are likely to not stick with it very long and end up giving up. Enjoy the process and you are more likely to lose the weight and keep it off.

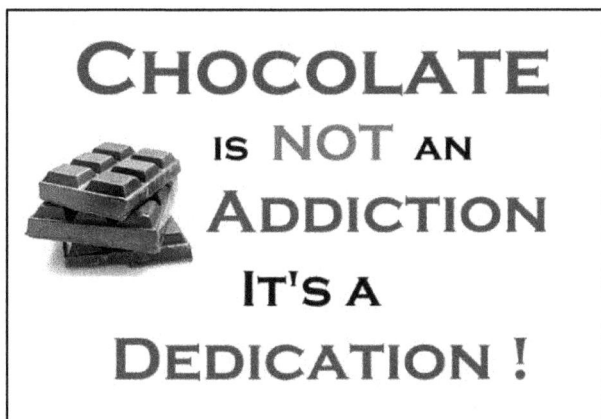

T-shirt design by Jack

Seconds

"If you want seconds, take a smaller portion first."

Weight loss is mostly a mental and emotional game. We have to find ways to help ourselves feel emotionally satisfied and think we've had enough. Taking a small portion in the first round is a smart move to allow yourself the feeling of indulging on seconds without really overdoing it. Take a tiny portion first and then let yourself have a second. If the first isn't that delicious, skip the second helping altogether.

Cookies

"I'll follow a chocolate chip cookie anywhere."

I have had to eliminate certain sugary foods, such as chocolate chip cookies, from my house. If I know they are within the walls of my home, my brain tells me, "Remember how good those taste? Go get some cookies." Doesn't matter if they are in the freezer. Frozen cookies taste great to me – I guess I have strong teeth. I simply can't have them around or I will eat them, and eat too many. Like Jack, I can follow them wherever we put them. I no longer bake them during the holidays, and I don't buy them very often. Keeping my home tempting-cookie free is very helpful to my efforts to not overindulge.

Another option suggested by Weight Watchers fellow member, Cheryl, is to prepare cookie dough and then freeze little unbaked rounds in two-cookie packages. She takes out just two at a time and fresh bakes them for herself. I admire Cheryl's commitment to herself to take the time to divide the raw dough into two-cookie portions so she can enjoy but not overeat. Losing weight does take effort. Cheryl's great idea allows her to enjoy cookies but with built-in limits.

Both options are good strategies if we can follow through long term. Choose a plan, and if you can stick to it, it's a good plan for you.

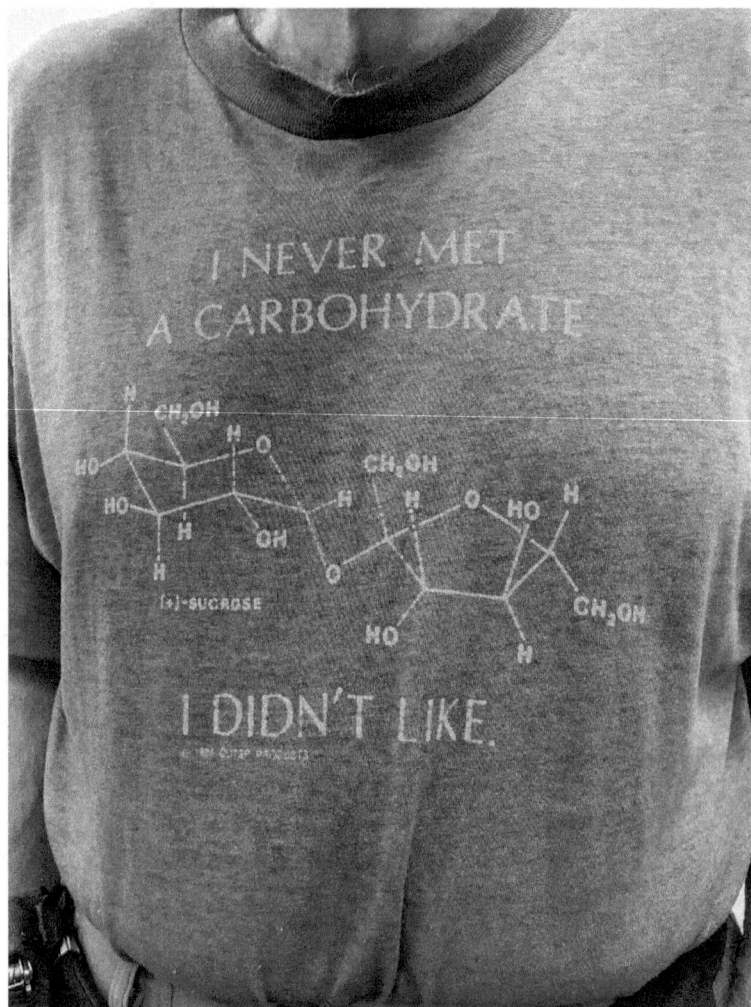

Holiday Helps

"At holidays, I stay away from the food by playing with my grandkids."

So often we focus on food at parties. What will we serve? What will we eat? One of my favorite ways to not overeat at a party is to focus on the people – focus on relationships. Make it about connecting with others, rather than just treating myself to food. And if there are kids present, they always welcome adults who want to play games with them, like hide-and-seek. It's a great way to enjoy relationships – not make it just about the food – and get some exercise in as well.

Deprivation

"Deprivation leads to bingeing."

One of the great things about Weight Watchers is that there is a way to eat nearly any food and still lose weight. Using the points system makes it possible. All foods are allowed. Each food has a points value, and every day we have a budget. As long as we stay within our budget, we are good. But even with this freedom, I have made the choice to not allow myself to eat some foods because their points value is so high. However, because I rarely give myself a chance to enjoy these foods, when I do have one, I tend to over indulge. For me, cookies and pizza fall into this special-food category. A better way is to learn to enjoy the foods I really love and have them more often. They lose their power when I do have them more often, and I have better success setting limits. Being on a "diet" means eliminating foods. Choosing a way of life means learning to have foods I love within limits and leads to long-term success.

On Changing a Routine

"When I started going to the gym after work, at first my family didn't like me coming home late. Then one day I skipped the gym and came home early. That threw them off because they weren't expecting me so soon. I learned then that your family will adapt when you change your schedule. So don't worry about their initial reaction when you change. They will adjust."

A good number of those of us with weight problems have difficulty putting ourselves first, especially when it comes to our weight loss. Jack made a change to his daily routine, which required an adjustment for his family. And they did adjust. I also had to learn to not sacrifice my need to eat healthy meals by catering to my own family's desire to eat more fattening dinners. I made a change and started cooking more healthy meals. At first, they complained about all the chicken, but I decided my health was more important and I needed to stay committed to my own journey. And besides, they knew how to make themselves a sandwich! A healthy lifestyle may mean we have to stand up for our own needs and let our loved ones have time to adjust. And in time, they do.

Enjoyable Workouts

"I reward myself when I work out by saving movies I want to watch for when I'm on my workout equipment, and then I watch them on my tablet."

I had my husband mount a TV in my workout room, and I find that watching favorite shows while I am on my recumbent bike makes the time fly by. Jack rewards himself for his workout time by saving movies for just when he's on his equipment. If what we do to move is pleasurable, we are much more likely to stick with it, obviously. I also enjoy sports as a way to move. For me that is golf, cross-country skiing, and bowling. To make my daily walk more pleasurable, I take my camera with me and search for beauty in my neighborhood as I walk. This makes the journey an artistic adventure. I also love to walk the mall, especially when I drift into a store and find a cool item I like. Shoe shopping is a great activity, if you ask me. The point is to find ways to move that we enjoy, and we will most likely consistently keep these activities as part of our long-term lifestyle.

Plateaus

"I was on a plateau. So I looked at my trackers on the weeks I lost weight and compared them to the plateau weeks. I figured out that during the weeks I lost, I didn't have dairy. So I reduced my dairy and started losing again. Dairy can cause inflammation, and it did for me."

Keeping your weekly trackers or looking back through your app food history is a very good way to learn about what you are doing, what really works, and what doesn't. I did this to find how many points a day I needed in order to lose. My own magic number. I shoot for that daily, and when I meet that number, I lose. Correlating what and how much I ate to whether or not I lost taught me that. For Jack, he learned that dairy stalls his weight loss. Another lady in my meetings learned she was eating too little fat to lose, and once she increased that she got past her plateau. So study the good and the not-so-good and learn what your body needs, and you will have more information to arm you in the weight loss battle.

Controlled Gluttony

"Sometimes you can choose controlled gluttony. Pick an end date for when you will stop enjoying something."

One of the great advantages to Weight Watchers is that there are no forbidden foods, and we are taught how to eat everything, including indulgent items. But we still can eat too much of them and lose control. So allowing a little rebellion and then setting a quit date is a smart way to not get stuck in an endless parade of calories into the mouth. I had leftover birthday cake in my house. I told myself I could have one piece each day for two days and then I had to quit. By then it had lost its luster anyway. I moved on and went back to healthier choices.

Skinny People

"There is nothing worse than a skinny glutton."

Those of us with lifelong weight issues do resent those who can just eat and eat and not gain weight. I remember an episode of Oprah where she complained to Dr. Phil about people who can eat so much and are still skinny. Dr. Phil's answer was, "Yeah, well, that's not you!" Yep, we need to let go of that difference. It doesn't help us any to have a pity party over having a slower metabolism. Get over it and own your body. This is the path we have been given. Accept that and learn. Everyone has a unique path in life. Live your path and become better through it.

Handling a Buffet – Strategy #1

"When I go to a buffet, the first thing I do is look at everything on the buffet and figure out what I really want, and skip the things I eat normally. Then I just take a small portion so I can take seconds if I want."

I have been using this great buffet strategy ever since Jack shared it in one of our Weight Watchers meetings. And it works. I find I enjoy the buffet, feel satisfied, and manage my intake well as a result. It also works for festivals. I check out all the vendors, decide what I really want to try, and skip foods that aren't special. Then I start with a small portion of what I thought looked good first. I recently did this for the Taste of Randolph Street in Chicago and had a loss the next day at my weigh-in. The strategy works!

Handling a Buffet – Strategy #2

"When I go to a buffet, I look over all the items and I pick three things which I would enjoy the most, and I have those. If one of those three turns out to not taste that good, I throw that out and pick the fourth-best thing."

I was at a family party yesterday, with a big spread of items to choose from, similar to a restaurant buffet. I remembered Jack's words and just chose the top three things that looked best to me. I had one fried chicken breast, the low-cal seven-layer salad, and the broccoli dish. I skipped having a chicken wing, the mostaccioli, and the potato salad. I was satisfied and just ate what tasted best to me. I let myself have a small scoop of ice cream for dessert, too. I was happy to see my weight stayed the same the next morning when I got on the scale. Jack's strategy helped me enjoy the food but not overindulge. Strategies like this add up to success.

Emotional Satisfaction

"If you are not emotionally satisfied after a meal you are going to keep on eating."

Just as distracted driving is dangerous to road safety, distracted eating is dangerous to weight loss success. Eating while watching TV, reading, driving, or playing with my phone all mean that I am not connecting to my food and that when I do this I am more likely to keep looking for more to eat after the meal. It's better to take in the enjoyment of the flavors and let myself know that I have eaten. Then I don't have the strong desire to keep eating after eating, allowing for better weight loss results.

Appetizers

"When we host a dinner we serve fruit as an appetizer."

In addition to fruit, I like to serve appetizers of shrimp cocktail, vegetables with low-fat dip, and deviled eggs made with low-fat mayonnaise. I have found that most of these items are appreciated by my family as well. And if others are hosting, I often will volunteer to bring one of these so I can guarantee I have something good for my weight loss plan to munch on while waiting for the main meal. We have to take the lead in our health. Plan to succeed.

Quitting

"The only way to fail is to quit."

When Jack said this to me I felt very encouraged because I had at that time gained back all of the weight I had lost, even though during the weight gain I had been faithfully attending meetings every week. I kept trying over and over. I was feeling like a failure, but I agree—if you never give up, you haven't failed. I haven't and I won't. Even if I keep blowing it, I am committed to never giving up. And that makes me a success at any weight.

Tracking

"When you track it, you own it."

Writing down my food transgressions does connect my brain to these actions. I do own it then. I find sometimes it's not as terrible as I made it in my mind, allowing me to get back to my plan faster. Ignoring the food by not tracking it causes me to essentially just eat without reining in my impulses. The act of writing it down (or entering it into a tracking app) helps me stop eating without any thought and helps me set and keep my necessary food limits. I own it.

Food Sharing

"Share your food. Let someone else wear it."

Just because there is food on my plate or on the table doesn't mean it has to be eaten by me. One way to deal with it without overeating is to offer it to others. This is especially important in restaurants that serve crazy large portions. I can share with others, or I can share it with myself at another time by splitting the meal and taking half home. Whoever eats it does wear it.

Feeling Sorry for Yourself

"Pity parties are well catered."

I'm one of those people that when trying to avoid feeling angry, anxious, or sad has the urge to self-comfort with food. I remember visiting my disabled mother and when I got home I wanted to eat a big bowl of ice cream, even though I was not hungry. As Jack liked to say, pity parties are well catered. A better choice was to listen to my needs and reach out to have them met. I really needed to call a friend and have them give me the mothering that Mom's limitations restricted her from providing. A party with a girlfriend is much better than a party with pity and too much ice cream.

Getting to Goal

"You have to look at getting to your goal weight not as an end, but as a new beginning."

Jack has been at his goal weight since 2000. He talks about setting new goals and new challenges for himself, to help him stay focused. He looked at the milestone of getting to goal as the start of a new adventure in learning to keep eating well and finding new positive goals to achieve, like hiking the Grand Canyon, which he did accomplish. Other goals could be to do a 5K, complete a half marathon or mini triathlon, lift heavier weights, or try a new recipe every week. All are ways to keep the energy focused on the journey of health. Goals can make every day a new beginning and can refresh our focus.

Alcohol Humor #2

"Vodka only counts as 60% water."

Not really. This was Jack being sarcastic.

My favorite mixed drink is what I call a Blueberry Vodka Mojito. Mix blueberry vodka, diet Sprite, fresh squeezed lime juice, mint, and crushed blueberries over crushed ice. I serve these drinks at parties, and I end up making a lot of them because people love them. Just portion each ingredient to your taste. And watch out, because they go down easy.

Hosting Holidays

"I like to host holidays because we have home court advantage."

Hosting does mean having control over the menu, allowing for healthy options that can help to support the weight loss effort. But sometimes when I host I miss this opportunity. Sometimes I throw weight loss out the window and just make things that will please my guests but not help me. But in reality, healthy food can taste delicious if cooked properly.

I like when my step-mom hosts because I know she makes healthy meals for holidays, and they always taste terrific. The point is to get together and enjoy each other anyway, not feast until we pass out. Offer to host and make weight-friendly dishes. The family still appreciates the meal.

Challenges

"Challenge yourself. When you do there are new opportunities."

New challenges do bring new opportunities. My company moved to a location over a mile from the train station in the city. The company provided a shuttle bus to get to and from the building and the train, but I challenged myself to walk the distance instead of taking the shuttle bus.

The first week of walking twice a day caused a lot of pain in my legs and feet. But I pressed on and stuck with it. Within a couple of weeks, the walk was no longer difficult, my jeans were looser, and I started enjoying everything I was seeing in the new neighborhood on my walk twice a day. The challenge gave me the opportunity to explore a new area of the city and find cool places to shop and dine. The walk gave me more life. The challenge gave me a new opportunity.

Winter

"The good thing about winter is chocolate doesn't melt in your car."

Ah, Jack and his love for chocolate. Keeping snacks in the car can be helpful if they keep me from picking up french fries in a drive-through line on the way home from work. However, for me, if a snack is in my car or at my desk at work, I will eat it. If I bring two snacks to work, by the end of the day they will both be gone. If I bring three snacks, they will all be gone as well. So, I only bring in the snack limit I have for one day and then I do better. And I don't store chocolate in my car, even in winter.

Routines

"Routines can become ruts. You have to change the routine to get out of the rut."

Being a creative person, I am easily bored. If I eat the same food day after day, I rebel. I have found that switching up my food choices on a daily basis keeps me interested and compliant. However, I have to have a set of options that are weight loss friendly, which can be a challenge. I have to balance variety with staying on plan. Figuring out variations to my daily habits takes time and energy, too. Even the action of figuring out new things to eat is a change and can help break me out of a rut. Bottom line is that it does take energy to lose weight. But I'm worth it.

Becoming a New Person

"You become a new person when you lose weight."

Although after losing weight you are much the same, much is also transformed. Many of those who have lost a lot of weight share that they feel more confident as a result. Confidence helps with relationships, work, and living life more fully. We don't just look different, we feel differently about ourselves, which affects how we relate to others. So, in a way, we do become a new person – a physically, emotionally, and mentally healthier person, usually with much improved self-esteem. It's worth the work to get there. Press on.

Fake Allergies

"When someone offers me something fattening that I don't want to eat, I tell them I'm allergic – I break out in fat."

I have also claimed to be allergic to certain foods at restaurants to be sure the waiter and chefs followed through on my special weight loss requests. I have claimed to be diabetic to be sure I get a no-sugar item like diet soda instead of soda with sugar. I have claimed to be allergic to butter to keep the staff from topping my food with their typical butter balls. But I love Jack's humorous claim even better. He makes the point without offending. We need to speak up on our own behalf and make sure we are taken care of by others. Our lives are worth it.

Discouragement

"You need to declutter your mind. When I get discouraged I now choose to not focus on the negative. Instead, I choose to be positive."

Disbelief is powerful. Thinking that the weight can't come off leads to the weight not coming off. I know; I have struggled with this lack of faith in myself for many years. I appreciate Jack's admonishment to let go of negativity and instead choose to believe in the positive. I can get this weight off. It is within my power. I will do this. I am deciding to accept that as truth and remove the clutter of past failures. Yesterday does not dictate what tomorrow will be. I get to make my own fresh, new choices. I choose health today.

Stubbornness

"Use your stubbornness as persistence towards your goal."

One of my biggest strengths is that I don't give up easily on many things, including my weight loss. I have been attending meetings weekly since 2001. At first, I lost most of the weight, over 70 pounds, and got within 20 pounds of my goal. Then I had two events overthrow my success. First, I had a hysterectomy, which modified my metabolism. I was no longer able to eat the same amount and lose. As a matter of fact, if I ate that amount I gained. Second, my husband was diagnosed with cancer. My life became much more stressful, and that stress lasted for many years, as we had a long battle. Meanwhile, I had to change jobs several times, and I had a heavy workload. My husband passed away in 2012.

On top of having a modified, slower metabolism, I chose to sooth my stress with my favorite vice, food. I ate without counting and gained back all the weight, plus added another 30 pounds, even though I was attending weekly Weight Watchers meetings the entire time. Attending the meetings didn't mean I was actually applying the inspiration to my life. I wasn't.

But I never gave up. I kept coming and kept trying new things. I just wouldn't give up. And I haven't.

I have remarried – a loving, healthy man. I have learned to have better boundaries with my work, my doctor has put me on thyroid medication, and I am now making progress towards getting back to my lighter self. Stubbornness is truly a great strength when applied to weight loss. Jack is right, as usual.

Habits

"It takes 20 days to form a habit. Except a bad habit."

It does seem much easier to form a bad habit than a healthy one. Part of that is because some foods cause cravings. For example, salty foods cause craving for more salty foods. Sugary foods cause cravings for more sugary foods. It may be easier to control these cravings if we reduce or eliminate these foods from our normal diet. What we need more than salt is water. And what we need more than sugar is fruit. Try replacing salty snacks with more water, and sugary ones with fruit, and see if the cravings are reduced. Might be a good new habit to form. Try that for 20 days and see if it can be part of your new lifestyle.

Getting Older

"I'm not putting on more weight as I get older. I just can't hold my breath as long."

I do work hard to camouflage my weight, sometimes wearing baggy clothes or just covering my especially troubling areas. But lately I have decided that I can be proud of how I look as I look today, with or without extra weight. I choose to stop feeling ashamed of myself as a large lady and instead do the best with what I have and wear it with pride. It's not true to tell myself that beauty is only thin and that until I obtain thin I can't be beautiful. I choose to believe all of us have beauty, no matter our size or wrapper. Embrace what we have and who we are today.

Handling High-Calorie Dishes

"When someone is serving a high-calorie dessert or dish and they want you to try it, have a few bites and then, say, 'Thank you, very delicious, I wish I could eat more but I'm full,' and then offer it to others. You can also ask to take it home or ask for the recipe."

I had a Greek grandmother who showed us her love by feeding us. Often, I would come home from school and on our kitchen counter or stove would be homemade apple pie or chicken soup that she'd brought over and left for us. I didn't care for the pot of cooked dandelion greens, however, but my dad ate it up like candy. It was her way of loving us.

When people at work bring in their special baked creations, they don't really want to hear, "No thank you. I'm trying to lose weight." Jack's response is kinder. Let them know you appreciate the work they did, their good baking, and so much so that you want to share it with others – a simple change in response that means the baked goods do not have to throw off our plan. Take a little, and then let others finish them off.

Accountability

"You have to own your actions."

When I don't write down what I eat and skip meetings, I get this general amnesia about what I am doing with my weight. I am not able to own what I am doing, because I don't even remember. Not only is there no progress, I always start gaining weight. Writing down what I eat and stepping on an official weigh-in scale allow me to own what I am doing and make real change.

Weight loss takes energy and work. The weight never magically falls off. I have to take an honest look at what I am doing, not make excuses for that but own that I have made those choices, and then I can make real changes so I can lose the weight. Another common Weight Watchers saying is, "If you bite it, write it." Own it.

Silly Song

My motivational song is "I Don't Look Good Naked Anymore," by the Snake Oil Willie Band.

Even if we lose all our weight and work out regularly, there is this reality that as we age gravity takes over and the body tends to change. Losing weight just to look good may be futile as we age. But hopefully as we age the reality of our health is more important, so that tends to be our new motivator.

At my age, while I would like to look better to the eye, I am even more concerned with causing unpleasant health issues for myself in my late years. Obesity increases the chances of so many health issues, including heart disease, diabetes, and some cancers. My first husband fought cancer and passed away from the disease. I know firsthand how not fun that road is. That fear is helping me to fight and care. I'd rather live my senior years enjoying life, not fighting health issues. Losing the weight increases that likelihood. Healthy is sexy, too.

Rapid Weight Gain

"We don't gain weight overnight, but it seems like it."

When I'm not writing down my daily consumption, I inevitably eat too much for my body to burn. And since I'm not spending any energy paying attention to my daily diet, time flies in my happy denial. A year can pass before I really stop my numbed happiness. Weight gain is guaranteed. It seems like it comes on in an instant because my mind is not part of my daily food intake process. In reality, weight gain is not overnight. It happens when we string together a set of days where we just pay no attention to what we are doing, so it seems to be a quick gain.

Losing weight does require attention. It seems to take longer, but it really doesn't. It just takes more focus, and change happens more slowly than we'd like. Stay patient and be persistent. We are worth the effort. Fight hard for you.

How to Fail

"The only way to fail is to quit."

I have been attending meetings weekly for over 17 years. At first, I lost most of my excess weight, but then I gained it back plus some, the whole time attending meetings and weighing in every week. I felt like a failure. I appreciated Jack's encouragement that I really hadn't failed because I never stopped coming and trying to re-motivate myself. If I'd walked away, then I would have failed. But I hadn't.

Favoring Parties

"During the holidays, I decide what parties I will attend and which I will skip, and plan my points accordingly. I plan ahead."

At my office we have essentially food fests during the holidays. Everyone brings in something yummy, and we spread it around a huge conference room. Most of it is decadent and bad for the body. The last few years I have avoided the room altogether. I found that I ended up with a full plate of little bites and had a hard time figuring out the damage and knowing how much I should eat on those days. Not all the items are worth the price, too, and I can end up feeling dissatisfied from these food events.

Other parties are easier to manage. My step-mom is health minded, so I know when I have a holiday meal at her house the food will be lightened up and good for the weight loss effort. Plus, she is family and super nice.

Some parties are just not worth it during the holidays. Let's pick the best for us in terms of both fun and physical health and live longer and happier.

Holiday Reward

"To get through the holidays, plan something you normally don't enjoy as a treat after the holidays."

When Jack shared this I said, "Oh, you mean like going shoe shopping?" He answered, "For me that would be torture."

Each of us enjoys different things. For me, getting a massage or shopping for clothes is a treat. Jack enjoys hikes in the woods as a special reward.

What a great idea to promise myself a reward if I stay on plan during the holidays. While I'm saying "no" to indulging, I am saying "yes" to a gift to myself after it's all over. This is a great way for us to not feel deprived as we avoid eating every cookie we meet during the holiday season.

This reward can also be a special type of food, like a favorite dessert, planned and measured out. Try making a deal with yourself. Say "no" to endless holiday indulging but promise yourself a special treat if you stick to your plan – and then give yourself the treat when you've fulfilled your promise.

Routine Warning

"When you eat or do the same things over and over, your routine can become a rut. Change the types of food you eat. Mix it up."

When I eat the same thing every day, my body does get used to the food and calorie level, and I often find my weight loss is stalled. The body responds to varied food types and amounts. Many people have said the way to break a plateau is to vary the number of points per day by even large amounts. It takes a different kind of discipline to do this, and it can be scary to have days where I intentionally eat way over or way under my points, but it does shake up the metabolism and does allow for losses to flow again. Variety is the spice of life and key to breaking out of ruts and plateaus.

Not a Good Idea

"If a man asks a woman to go to Weight Watchers with him, it's suicide."

My Weight Watchers leader asked us to invite people to our open house. Jack's response was the above. He wasn't going to dare indicate to one of his female friends that she needed to come to a meeting. He figures it's not a good move to tell a woman she needs to lose weight!

It does need to be our own idea to try to lose weight. No one else can do it for us.

But, when I was 18 and weighed 223 pounds, two ladies I worked with invited me to attend Weight Watchers with them. At first, I was embarrassed that they'd asked me, but then I decided to give it a try. I lost over 70 pounds on the program. I'm so thankful they did take the risk to invite me. And I enjoyed attending the meetings and working on my weight with these inspirational ladies. Inviting others can work out to be a very good idea as long as you're not Jack attempting to ask out a lady by inviting her to a meeting.

The Grand Canyon

Jack said his daughter agreed to hike the Grand Canyon with him because she figured she could find some guys with great bodies there.

Finding ways to get our family members to be active with us can be a challenge. When I got married my husband was not a golfer, but I was. I found the way to get him into the sport was to plan golf with a good friend of his and his wife, and buy a lot of beer. My husband then connected learning golf to a lot of laughs, instead of just being a chore.

Jack's daughter decided that hiking the Grand Canyon with her dad was a chance to meet guys who were in shape. They did hike that huge crater and created a great father–daughter memory in doing so.

Our family members want to support us, but sometimes we have to be creative to get the follow-through for what we need. Bribes work.

Treats at Work

Jack: "When a person brings in treats to work, I have a couple bites, tell them how delicious it is, and say that I want to save the rest for dessert after lunch."
Meeting member: "Do you eat it then?"
Jack: "No, unless it's chocolate."

Jack loves chocolate like no one I've ever known. He even has designed his own T-shirts proclaiming his love for chocolate and wears them often to Weight Watchers meetings. And he lost his weight enjoying chocolate nearly every day. He just budgeted his daily points allocation so he could enjoy his favorite food. The Weight Watchers points system allows for any and all foods. We have a daily budget for spending points that we have to live within. We can include what we love, and those who do eat what they love, do better. The problem for me is I don't have just one food I love. So I have applied Jack's method to all of them – have those treats but count them in my daily points budget. I did this when I lost 73 pounds on the plan. You can stick to a plan if it includes the foods you love while reining them in. Try eating one special thing you love every day but count the points and eat within your limit. Make it your special daily treat. And this will be a lifestyle you can maintain, not a short-term diet you can't maintain.

"On weigh-in day I just eat all my points in chocolate."

Insights from Other Meeting Members
From Cheryl

Peace with Food

"You can have a war with food, or you can say to food, 'OK, let's work together'."

Cheryl has lost over 158 pounds on Weight Watchers in the past 10 years and continues to attend weekly meetings, sharing insights and helpful ideas each time.

One way I was at war with food was by eliminating foods I loved, causing me to feel deprived. Another was to throw out the tracker and indulge without counting, and then gain weight. In both cases I was battling food instead of finding a way to be at peace.

Working with food and not against it means planning for the foods I love and letting me have them, but measuring the portions and counting the points as part of my daily plan. Another way is to find a substitute for foods I love that satisfies my desires but doesn't sabotage my efforts. A third option is to find a pleasurable activity to focus on instead of food. All of these are choices that work together with food, instead of being at war with such a basic, daily need. Finding a way to make this a peaceful process means it can be sustained and I can do this long term. Negotiation wins over battles. I have found a way to negotiate this so that my desires and my weight loss efforts both win.

The Three Bite Rule

"Whenever I am tempted to eat something that I shouldn't have too much of, I use the Three Bite Rule."

Cheryl's explanation of her Three Bite Rule is based on her observations of herself. The first bite of a decadent food is the best. The flavors are most pronounced and affective to the palate. The second bite is good but doesn't give the full impact that the first bite gave. The third bite is also good, but the flavor is not nearly as powerful. At that point, the subsequent bites do not provide the flavor boosts the first three bites gave, and it's easier to stop. Cheryl remembers this when faced with something she wants but knows she needs to not have much of. She follows her Three Bite Rule – just have three bites and then stop. She finds she is able to stop, but she doesn't feel deprived because she did get to enjoy some of the special treat. The rule has helped Cheryl have success.

From Judy

One Week at a Time

"Focus on one week at a time. You can do anything for one week."

Judy is another very insightful woman in our weekly meetings who has lost 30 pounds and been at her goal weight since March 2015. She comes nearly every week to meetings and encourages us often with her wisdom.

Judy is so right that changing behavior by focusing on just the week ahead is easier for our minds to commit to than trying to tell ourselves this is for a longer period, even though it is.

I find that making a week-long commitment and setting my weekly meeting as the checkpoint works for me, helping me to stay on plan. It's true – we can do anything for just a week. Then if we string together these weeks, the next thing we know is that we've stuck to our new way of life longer and we are heathier and happier. One week at a time is key.

Adjustments

"When I am changing something in what I normally eat, I ask myself, 'Is this something I would do if I weren't trying to lose weight?' If not, make a different adjustment so it is a new long-term lifestyle, not a temporary diet."

I just love this wisdom from Judy. So smart. Sometimes we try too hard to lose weight. We make it a "diet" that we can't sustain. One example for me was eating the same selection at the same place every day for lunch because I saw that I was able to lose weight when I did this. But I am not the type of person who likes eating the same thing every day. That is something I would never do if I weren't trying to lose weight, so that means it isn't a sustainable solution for my weight loss effort. I need to find choices I can do for the long term.

I have also done this by trying to eat some food selections I just plain do not love, such as TV dinners. I would much rather eat my own home cooking than a TV dinner. If I do have one, I have to supplement the frozen food with a fresh salad or fruit or I feel deprived.

Food should be delicious, especially when we're trying to lose weight. As long as the portions are down, we can enjoy just about anything.

From Donna

Rabbit Food

"I've been eating so much lettuce lately I'm hopping like a bunny."

I chuckled as Donna shared this in our meeting one week. Donna was struggling with the program. Sure, vegetables are low in calories, fat, and points and high in nutrients, but if that's all we eat, we can find that we miss other foods and rebel. Moderation is needed even with healthy foods. Our bodies and minds do better with a variety of foods. So mix it up.

From Susan

Sneakers

"I'm so bad at running, I'm like a brick with sneakers on."

I tried jogging for two days about 25 years ago. Bouncing my large, overweight body up and down on my toes was too much torture for me. Like Susan, I felt like I was wearing brick sneakers. I reverted to walking or riding my recumbent bike, both of which are a lot easier on my joints while providing great value to my body. We have to find the activity that works with who we are in order to succeed.

From Carla

Brownies

"We don't want brownies to go bad, but we don't feel disappointed when a vegetable goes bad."

How true is Carla's observation on how sugar-prone and vegetable-averse we tend to be. I'm not sure why, but I've always liked vegetables, even as a child. Maybe my mom really knew how to make them taste good. And I still love them today. The only exception is cooked dandelions, which my Greek grandmother used to bring to our house regularly. I tried them once, but their bitter taste was not pleasant to my palate. My dad inhaled them as if they were candy, or brownies.

When I was a child, sometimes my best friend would invite me over for dinner with her family. I used to watch her fight with her parents over her refusal to eat her green beans and I'd think, "Just give me a fork. I'll take care of those for you." But her parents demanded they go into my friend's little frame, not mine. She has never had a weight problem, and I have struggled with my weight my entire life. Maybe being a picky eater is a blessing.

Like my mother, as an adult I have learned how to cook vegetables so they taste great. Daily I enjoy all the powerful benefits they provide – nutrients, fiber, filling me up, and so much more. I still don't let the veggies go bad.

Carla joined Weight Watchers in 2017 and has lost over 20 pounds so far.

From Crystal

Monthly Challenges

"Every month I give myself a new challenge. This month I gave myself the challenge of giving up chips because I was eating too many of them."

I was very inspired when I heard Chrystal share this in one of our Weight Watchers meetings. Setting new challenges is such a great way to keep my energy focused on my mission. Here are some goals I have set for myself:

1. Track 100% for seven days.
2. Drink half my weight in ounces of water every day for a week.
3. Give up caffeine for a month.
4. Give up sugar for a month.
5. Do 30 minutes on my recumbent bike a day for at least five days this week.

Although the Weight Watchers plan doesn't include such "rules," those goals can help the body to both burn better and work better. Keep changing it up and making it fresh and new.

From Joe

Small Goals

"I set a small goal that I have a good shot of making."

I have found that I have been able to consistently follow through on a goal if it's a small one, rather than a grandiose plan. My first recent goal was just to track everything I ate, not to necessarily change what I was eating, just write it all down. After two weeks of successful tracking, I added increasing my activity to several more days a week. After a couple of weeks of making these practices my new routine, I added trimming down my daily intake by just a few hundred calories, or about five points a day. Later I added increasing my water intake. Then I added attending a second meeting workshop during the week. Each goal was a small one I knew I had a good chance of achieving. Small goals added up to a big difference. I was healthier and lost weight.

Joe joined Weight Watchers in April 2019 and has lost 15 pounds so far.

From Margie

Move

"When I'm too tired to move, I tell myself to move so I won't be so tired."

I recently gave up caffeine to help improve my sleep, which did help. I also found that eliminating caffeine benefited me all day long. I was calmer and felt less stressed, and my skin looked better due to improved hydration. When I woke up feeling a little groggy, instead of drinking coffee I jumped onto my recumbent bike for a half hour or took a walk. I found the activity woke me like a cup of coffee used to, but without all those other negative side-effects. Exercise does generate energy, and of course it does a whole lot more, including helping to accelerate weight loss. If I can't take a nap to help with tiredness, I do the opposite – get busy moving!

Margie joined Weight Watchers in January 2019 and has lost 16 pounds so far.

From Jodie

Workout Limitations

"You can't work off a bad diet."

Jodie is my current Weight Watchers workshop leader. She's pretty amazing. Jodie is quite energetic, positive, wise, and skilled at helping people share their insights with the others. And she makes us laugh nearly every meeting. She is very loved by our group, and I find that meetings she leads are very motivating for me.

Jodie lost 75 pounds on Weight Watchers and has kept if off since June 2016. She now works not only as a Weight Watchers leader, but also as a fitness coach in a gym. She is a great example to us of what it means to be committed to health.

I have heard a lot of people say their plan to take off excess weight was to just exercise more. In Jodie's work as a trainer, she has seen firsthand how workouts alone don't usually succeed if a person continues to eat as they did when they put on the weight. What we eat and how we eat are vital components of weight loss. Working out alone is not likely to succeed for long-term health. To successfully get off excess weight and be healthy, we need to do both: eat better and move our bodies.

Self-Talk

"Stop listening to yourself and start talking to yourself."

After Jodie made this statement in our meeting she explained that we will be more successful if we stop listening to negative and critical self-thoughts and start telling ourselves positive and loving thoughts. For example, I got on my scale today and saw a two-pound gain. I thought, "What did I do to cause that?" And I remembered that last night I tried a new "low-cal" ice cream, but I knew it was really not that low cal. I knew it was too much for me, and I'm pretty sure it turned into weight over the evening while my body tried to figure out what to do with the fatty, sugary treat so close to bedtime. Instead of thinking negative thoughts such as "I will never lose this weight" or "I was so stupid to do that; I should have known better," I told myself, "OK, I learned that I can't get away with indulging in that type of ice cream without a weight gain hit. I need to not eat that brand anymore and to stick to the better items I know don't cause that issue." I told myself a loving, positive plan to improve myself and just kept right on going with my efforts to make better food choices. Positive, practical self-talk is a great tool for success.

Mindfulness

"That's showing mindfulness."

I realized that I have really been eating at a maintenance level, not really at a weight loss level. I figured that I needed to shave off some points per day if I was going to lose. I decided to plan out my points at the beginning of the day so I could be sure I had enough left to have an evening snack but stay within a better limit. I know I am more successful if I plan a low-points evening snack than if I try to white-knuckle resist the temptation to snack. But if I don't plan out my points, I end up eating too much for the day to lose anything. After I began this track-and-plan-ahead strategy, I began losing again. I shared my new plan in my Weight Watchers meeting. My leader, Jodie, pointed out to the group that this was an example of mindfulness. I'd thought about what was really going on for me, what was keeping me stuck, and what I could do to modify my daily routine in order to be more successful at weight loss. It pays to take the time to think through what we are doing and how we can make it better.

From Louann

Getting Back on Track

"You can go back on plan as soon as you brush the crumbs off your face."

Slipups are a normal part of the typical weight loss journey. This quote from my former Weight Watchers leader is one of my favorites – I use it after a slipup to remember I can get back to my plan immediately. Forgive and restart. If I don't, I find myself slipping from a bad moment to a bad week. Instead, I remember to brush off the crumbs and start again.

From Jeff and Alexandra

Budgeting

"Going on Weight Watchers is like going on a food budget."

There are nutritional "bills" you are required to pay, just like your electricity bill, your gas bill, etc. You have to eat fruit and vegetables, protein, healthy fat, and dairy to keep things running smoothly. Then you have so much currency (points) left over for fun stuff, but there is still a daily limit.

When you are overweight, it's like you are in weight debt. You've spent too much. I was in financial debt before, and the way I got out of debt was to cut back my spending to a bare minimum and just patiently wait for the funds to come in to reduce the debt. The same process works with weight loss: that is, I need to adopt a lower and slower food spend rate and be patient. The weight debt (the pounds) will drop.

Jeff has lost over 60 pounds on Weight Watchers since joining in January 2018.

From Me (my Weight Watchers buddies encouraged me to share these with you)

Distraction Plan

"When I am tempted to eat when I'm not really hungry, I invoke my Overeating Distraction Plan."

When I'm tempted to eat something I don't need that will interfere with my weight loss, I invoke my distraction list. This is a list of things I enjoy doing and can go do instead of eating. Distraction is a powerful mental plan. Below is my list. Jack says item #5 is torture for him. We each have to make our own list of self-giving things to do instead of eating. If I can't do any of these activities at the time, I just find something else to do to distract my mind from the temptation. I have found that this works especially well if I am tempted to eat when not hungry, which is likely an emotional eating situation. I used to think I had to find a food substitute or the desire would not go away. But then I learned that I didn't have to eat for the desire to be relieved. Action also relieves these desires and puts them to bed. Distraction is a powerful weight loss tool.

1. Play piano or guitar.
2. Write more stories.
3. Sit in my massage chair.
4. Watch a great TV show or movie.
5. Shop online for shoes or clothes.
6. Plan a party or dinner out with friends.
7. Look up low-point foods I can enjoy at restaurants.

My Metabolism Doesn't Read

"My metabolism doesn't read my tracker."

I have found that sometimes I want to not be completely honest with my points tracker journal or app when I track what I have eaten. But my body will not lose weight faster if I don't write it down. My metabolism doesn't read my tracker or log in to my Weight Watchers app. It "reads" what I give it, and that is it. My body is not fooled. After I came to this realization I decided it was just better to be completely honest with myself when I track. Honest tracking helps me know when I'm going over my daily allocation. If I gain weight, I can find the reasons in my tracker and then make the necessary adjustments.

Being a Hypocrite

"I'm a Weight Watchers hypocrite."

I realized one week that I am like a person who hears a sermon in church, agrees with the preacher, and then walks out and doesn't apply a single word of it to her life. I can often do this with my Weight Watchers meetings. I agree with all the good thoughts shared, I think of a way to make the next week better, I tell myself I'll do just that, and then I don't apply any change to my week. I'm like a Weight Watchers hypocrite. Once I realized this, I told myself if I want to actually lose weight, I have to actually do my plan. Then I started making traction.

Reality

"You have to deal with your reality."

A lady in our meeting shared about her struggle with following the program. She was a nurse who traveled to homes to administer care. She needed to pick up lunch for some of her clients, but her schedule only allowed her enough time to run through fast-food drive-throughs. She was getting her own lunch there as well, but not making good choices. Cheryl, who had lost over 150 pounds on Weight Watchers and often provided very helpful advice to the rest of us, suggested, "Why not go to the places which have something you like and is weight loss friendly?" Telling the nurse to not go to fast-food restaurants would not work for her life. Her reality was that she needed to do this for her work. So instead, we encouraged her to deal with her reality by continuing to go through fast-food drive-throughs but to make choices there that would be better for her weight loss efforts.

I work a full-time job in the city and live in the suburbs. When I come home from my long commute, I am tired and hungry. I found that if I tried to cook dinner, I ended up spending most of my night cooking, eating, and doing the dishes. I was having no life. I then chose to deal with this reality better. I changed to cooking meals on weekends and on the days when I work from home, and I made double of what we needed so I could freeze ready-to-eat meals for those long-commute days. The problem was solved. I found a way to make it work with my reality.

Fighting the reality of life isn't going to be a successful strategy. We have to find a way to make it work in the world we live within. Then we can succeed.

From Many of My Weight Watchers Buddies

Befriending Yourself

"Treat yourself as a friend."

I've heard many people say this in Weight Watchers meetings over the years. I haven't been very successful at following this advice until lately. Most of my life I have focused on the needs of others and neglected my own. It's my natural first response to most situations.

But lately I've been thinking of how I would treat me if I were a friend of mine. I ask myself, "How can I be nice to my friend Alexandra? What does she really like? What really makes her happy?" That helps me think of practical ways to be kinder to myself. For Christmas this year, my answer was, "Alexandra would like to get some beautiful brooches for Christmas because she loves those and collects them." I went out and bought myself a couple of inexpensive pieces of jewelry and will put those in my stocking to pretend Santa brought them for me. Sounds silly, but I've been looking forward to Christmas morning when I get to receive my new jewelry from "secret" Santa Alexandra. I do the same thought process with my meal choices. I think, "What does Alexandra like to eat? What is good for her body and her soul?" And then I let her have what she wants within healthy limits. Self-care is key for successful weight loss.

www.ingramcontent.com/pod-product-compliance
Lightning Source LLC
Chambersburg PA
CBHW062151020426
42334CB00020B/2557